This Workbook belongs to:

To download more free printable **Worksheets**, go to:

go.yogatrainersworkshop.com/sequencingsheets

Copyright © 2020 Julie Chavanu | Yoga Trainers Workshop
All Rights Reserved.

Sequencing Introduction

Creating a good class sequence is a very important aspect of teaching a yoga class.

Regardless of the reason people have come to yoga, if they are in an asana class, they are there for the work yoga does for their body: working out the kinks from the day, a bit of detoxing, building strength, gaining flexibility and best of all, Savasana.

To help your students get all they can out of their physical yoga practice, your sequencing needs to be thoughtful and take them progressively from pose to pose.

To support you as a teacher, this sequencing method and framework gives you a place to start when you plan your classes. If you teach regular classes, you'll be planning them frequently! Also, if you teach regular classes, your students will expect consistency from you and having a framework to rely on helps you give them that consistency. There are other benefits both you and your students will gain when you have a framework from which to begin creating great classes, read on!

Sequencing Classes

"Begin where you are." T.K.V. Desikachar

When designing a yoga class, the practice should be designed to accommodate a variety of student levels.

What does this mean? For a teacher, it means being prepared and have ready, modifications for the variety of students who may be in class. It may simply mean being prepared to offer modifications for the postures you've planned, or it may mean altering the flow of the entire sequence to accommodate the students who are in your class on a given day.

It doesn't mean that a class posted as a beginner class needs to be perfectly modified for an advanced student. Nor does it mean that a class billed as an advanced class needs to be perfectly adjusted for a beginner. It simply means to be prepared for a variety of students and address their needs the best you can.

The ideal <u>result</u> of any practice is to have been a tool in helping students feel better and for them to leave class with an increased sense of balance, openness and energy.

> "A complete and effective yoga class is one that allows students to progress steadily and simply from one place to another in their personal practice." -Mark Stevens

How? There are two main concepts to consider: Vinyasa Krama and Parinamavada.

When designing a practice for a class, one-on-one session or your own practice, the first concept to consider is that of Vinyasa Krama which in Sanskrit means the *logical sequencing of a practice*.

Applying Vinyasa Krama means being clear about the different aspects of the asanas you want to emphasize in class and that you prepare your students for postures gradually and in a way that reduces or negates undesired effects.

Vinyasa/Flow and Hatha Yoga classes that follow a simple progression are using the concept of Vinyasa Krama. The exact postures may vary in every class, but should build on one another, moving from simple to complex: Centering/Breathing, Active Practicing, Focusing, Deeper Stretching and Relaxing/Meditating.

What does it mean to sequence logically? For example, a teacher may choose to teach a class focused on hip-openers. To do so means paying attention to the logical progression of postures and how they are related to the hips. A teacher doesn't jump in and instruct backbends as one of the first postures. Instead, the teacher begins with warm-ups such as moving through Surya Namaskara (Sun Salutations) with lunges to bring heat and flexibility to the body, including balancing poses such as Dancers Pose and then moving to Pigeon on the floor. After this type of prep, backbends can be sequenced in.

We will cover each one of the sections in detail, putting the most emphasis on the asana section.

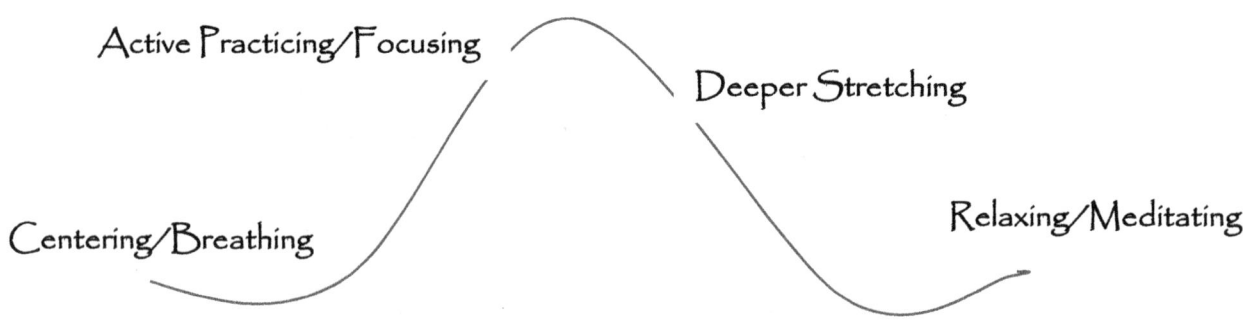

The second concept is *Parinamavada*, or the idea that life is in a constant state of flux, which is really at the core of the yoga philosophy and tradition. Inherently, we know this and in some areas of life, we easily accept it. In asana practice, as we teach, there are things we teachers can do to help our students apply it in class, too, such as offering modifications and reducing the number of postures we introduce in a class.

Sequencing a Yoga Class (5 stages of a class)
Centering/Breathing (1st stage)
Centering is a transition from the busy outside world, to our inner worlds, a chance to remember who we are and to practice from that place of authenticity. We can quiet the everyday chatter, re-focus our energy on healing, get calm and get a sense of our own body.

Take this time to encourage students to form an intention. Examples of intentions are:

- Be present here

- Put aside problems and worries
- Let the practice serve you
- Allow forgiveness
- Be compassionate to yourself
- Find balance
- Remember to breathe
- You might even read a *short* quote, one or two sentences (but keep it short!).

Don't get distracted though from getting the asanas going, that's why students are there!

Centering Practice Examples:
- ✓ Mountain pose – Mountain pose creates a tall posture and open space in which to focus on the breath and expand into the entire body. An option is to have students start with the hands at heart center and rock their body weight forward and back in the feet (slow movements).

- ✓ Child's Pose – A full-body resting pose that slows down the heart rate. The pose is geared to keeping your focus inward and restoring your energy. This is a great pose for an end-of-day centering practice to allow time for students to slow thoughts and bring awareness into the room and into their practice.

- ✓ Easy-Seated pose –Like it's name, it should be easy. Offer a blanket or rolled mat to sit on to elevate hips, allowing the inner thigh muscles and hips to relax. This sitting pose is frequently done in breathing and meditation practices. The key to getting comfortable in this pose is using your core (front/back/sides) to support you, so using props to establish that feeling can be very helpful to your students.

- ✓ Rag Doll: Another inward-turning pose, standing with feet hip distance apart, knees bent, standing in a very loose forward fold. Arms hanging at the floor or hands holding onto opposite elbows. Because the knees are generously bent, students will notice that the muscles of their legs work quite a bit in this pose and will begin to warm.

- ✓ Savasana: Starting where you plan to end can make for a great option. Anyone who's been to class before knows the relaxation of Savasana and it can trigger that sense of relaxing right from the start. It's a great accompaniment to breath-awareness as students can easily place a hand on their belly to monitor their breath. Before coming out, you can have students draw their knees in toward them and/or hold a knee in each hand and circle their knees to release their low back.

Breathing (continuation of 1ˢᵗ Stage)

After centering for a few minutes, the natural progression takes you into more intentional and aware breathing. Centering allows us to quiet our minds and come into a more focused awareness of our breath. This can take time to cultivate because our minds – certainly toward the beginning of any class – can be full of chatter and restlessness.

At this stage of class, simple awareness and a few moments to deepen breathing is ideal to get students started.

Active Practicing (2ⁿᵈ Stage)

This is where the magic of linking breath and movement really shows up!

A yoga practice should be balanced between rest and activity, it should be sensible and well structured (Vinyasa Krama), and as Patanjali so very briefly states in the Yoga Sutras, *steady and a good fit/comfortable*. A well-rounded practice should move a student through a wide range of motion, creating harmony within their bodies: bones, muscles, joints and organs.

Gentle warm-up exercises will ease the body into readiness. We should begin with simple poses and progress to the more difficult ones. A practice can start with movement that bends the body forward naturally or those in which we raise our arms or legs, *but a practice shouldn't begin with backbends or twists. Other poses to avoid in the beginning of practice are headstands, triangle, bow or plow.*

Active-Start Alternatives

Many times, a flowing or vinyasa sequence starts with Sun Salutations, however, there are certainly other asanas you can add to your sequence before you begin flowing in a more dynamic way. These could be added for beginner-flow or vinyasa classes or for more hatha-focused classes where you aren't practicing any/as many Sun Salutations. This is obviously not an all-inclusive list, but a place to start.

- ✓ Core-Warming:

    - From Savasana, students can do a variation of 'legs up the wall', but without a wall. When you bring legs up over hips, your core engages. You can have students shift legs forward/back and side to side in small movements that bring core awareness.

    - From Standing, students can come to Down Dog for an extended hold. This warms the entire body but can be core-focused. If they bend knees deeply (hovering off the floor) and almost in Table, the core focus is stronger still. You can flow students between the two, being mindful of not over-doing it with the wrists. Taking a break in Child's pose as needed.

- ✓ Half Vinyasas: If you start in a standing position for centering, you can work with breath/movement connection with this modification of Sun Salutations. Instead of stepping or jumping back to Chaturanga, skip that piece and come right back up to standing on an inhale. Repeat.

- ✓ Table/Cat/Cow: If you start in Child's pose, coming to Table and doing a few rounds of Cat/Cow connects breath to movement and gets low back muscles and joints moving. From here, you can move students to Down Dog and either Sun Salutations or Standing poses (for Hatha-focused classes).

Focusing (3rd Stage)

The introduction of balancing postures helps students move deeper into their practice and deeper into the balance between their mind and body. Focus is cultivated here. As we hold balance postures, our mind may race and our muscles may want to quit. By bringing our focus to the pose and our breathing, we can move past these distractions and *move beyond the concept of quitting*. Students have an opportunity to settle in to a calm (sometimes sweaty!) confidence about their abilities.

A simple way to begin tapping into deeper focus is through the practice of **drishti**. A gazing point *sends soothing messages to your nervous system* by reducing your visual distractions and settling your eyes.

Deeper Stretching (4th Stage)

Releasing occurs in a yoga practice most apparently as we move into deeper stretching. Beginning a class with breath awareness, those deep full inhalations and exhalations work to replace old energy with renewed energy. The powerful, focused breathing done in the Active and Focus sections of the practice helps heat the body, relax muscles and release old energy.

It is during this section in the practice, after your class has taken time to deepen their breathing, warm their muscles and focus their minds that you can take them through the deeper stretching poses. For many of your classes, this is the time when students come to the floor for poses such as forward folds, hip stretches (such as Pigeon) and deeper back bending. This can also be the time your students work the 'theme' pose of the class.

Relaxing (5th Stage)

Some classes may use Savasana as a meditation, but *the two are different*. Savasana allows the body to completely relax, and once we have reached this point in the practice where our body is open, tension has lessened and the mind is cleared of clutter, we can transition into our Savasana relaxation.

Most yoga classes incorporate Savasana at the end of class using this pose for relaxation. In Book 1, Sutra 34, Savasana is described as "lying flat on the ground, like a corpse. It removes fatigue and gives rest to the mind." One of my teachers often reminded us to *acknowledge all the good we'd done for ourselves in class* and to let our bodies be heavy as we took it all in.

Other Class Considerations
As you work through your class sequence, there are other things that teachers need to consider for their students, and they are just as important as the sequence itself! These considerations pull both from the idea of Vinyasa Krama as well as from Parinamavada. Having these available as a part of your logical sequence is important because of the fluctuations in our lives and bodies.

*Modifications
When working with the asanas, <u>be familiar with at *least one to two variations (or levels) and one to two ways to modify*</u> the posture for students who cannot execute the full pose.

*Counterposes
In yoga we use counterposes to *balance the possible negative effects of asanas*. Proper practice is not just a matter of advancing step by step to a certain pose or to the end of practice.

*Transitions
Injuries can occur when transitioning from one pose to another; coming into and out of a pose. Mostly, students are trying to move too fast or are eager to get out of a pose and lose the sense of mindfulness they established when coming into the pose.

*Rest
Obviously, we need a rest whenever we become out of breath or are no longer able to control our breath. Regardless, if our breath remains quiet and regular, we must still honor the fact that certain parts of our body will become tired or sore and need a rest. *If you need a break, take a break – and learn to observe that need in your students.*

Another Sequencing Concept: Reduce, Reuse, Recycle
In our classes, we strive to help students gain greater awareness of their bodies and to find some rest at the end of the movements. Sometimes though, in our eagerness to create new and unique class sequences, we forget that.

Our desire to create unique classes comes sometimes from our concern that our students will become bored in class by practicing the same postures over and over. Sometimes, this concern comes from our own boredom of teaching the same postures over and over.

Remind yourself that everyone's life is in flux – constant change or parinamavada – and many times the consistency of a yoga series (not just attending a regular class, but the actual consistency of a sequence) becomes a valuable tool for students to be able to gauge how those life fluctuations affect them physically. This is a uniting or yoking of body and mind, the very definition of yoga.

Reduce, reuse, recycle also gives us teachers an opportunity to find balance in our classes, preventing them from become overloaded with too many postures and too much for our students to process.

Active Class Section Sequence Examples

Active Practice section (Warrior 2 focus):

2 Rounds of Sun Salutation A
2 Round of Sun Salutation B

Vinyasa to Warrior 1 (hold each 5 Breaths) > Warrior 2 > Side Angle > Warrior 2 > Triangle. (Vinyasa to switch sides) Do this sequence 2x.

Vinyasa to Warrior 2 > Reverse Warrior > Warrior 2 > Crescent > Humble Warrior. (Vinyasa to switch sides) Do this sequence 2x.

Return to Mountain pose.

Active Practice section (Crescent Pose focus):

3 Rounds of Sun Salutation A
1 Round of Sun Salutation B

Vinyasa to Warrior 2 > Crescent pose > Crescent Twist > Side Angle. (Vinyasa to switch sides) Do this sequence 2x.

Vinyasa to Crescent > Crescent core > Crescent at 45 degrees > Lizard. Vinyasa to switch sides) Do this sequence 2x.

Return to Mountain pose.

Full Class Sequence Example

When you start as a new teacher, take more time when designing your classes. Sometimes it's helpful to *"pick a theme"* and work around it, such as hip-openers, heart-openers, upper body strengthening or backbends.

Using the same matrix outlined earlier (centering, breathing, releasing, etc) below is a basic outline for a themed class.

> **Shoulder Opener Class Example:**
> *Centering/Breathing – Sukhasana with Ujjayi Breath
> *Active Practicing
>   -Inhale arms wide, exhale to Anjali mudra (hands at heart-center)
>   -Surya Namaskara A and/or B: 1-4 cycles
>   -Table/cat/cow
>   -Downward Dog
>   -Plank, Side plank/both sides, Down Dog
>   -Warrior 1, Warrior 2, Reverse Warrior, Pyramid
>   -Switch sides (add Vinyasa)
> *Focusing – Side Angle (add bind as an option)
>   -Dancer, Uttansasana, Eagle
>   -Switch sides
> *Deeper Stretching – Half Bow on each side
>   -Full Bow, Child's pose
>   -Thread the Needle Twist
>   -Child's pose
>   -Bridge or Wheel
>   -Shoulder stand, Plow, Fish, Reclined Twist
> *Relaxing
>   -Savasana and Meditation

Notice how the practice started slowly and gently with easy postures designed to heat up the chest and shoulder areas. Then the practice progressed to postures that released any tension brought into the area from the deeper work. Suitable counter poses were used, along with the appropriate progression from gentle to difficult, creating a well-rounded practice.

How to use the Class Sequence Worksheets:

Using the concepts from the information above, use the worksheets to play with and create different class sequences. Use pencil and get a good eraser! Practice your created sequences on your own and see how they flow and how they make you feel.

Mix/match the sections across different classes to create more sequences, being mindful of preparing physically for different theme/peak poses.

Then, test them out in your classes.

When you attend classes, make notes about what you liked and how you can incorporate those ideas into your sequences.

There is a space at the end of each worksheets for Teacher Notes. The best way to find and develop your own teaching voice with your sequences is to make these kinds of notes. You'll then have created a resource to look back upon as you teach.

Start creating your own library of sequences!

Frame for a Class Sequence

Asana Examples

Centering/Breathing
- Childs
- Rag Doll
- Easy Seated
- Mountain

Active Practicing
- Sun Salutations
- Warriors & Variations

Focusing
- Tree
- Eagle
- Warrior 3
- Dancer's
- Arm Balances

Deeper Stretching
- Standing Forward Folds
- Seated Forward Folds
- Backbending

Relaxing/Meditating
- Savasana
- Easy Seated
- Pranayama

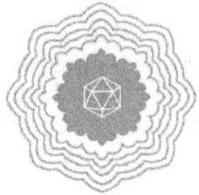

Class Sequence Worksheets

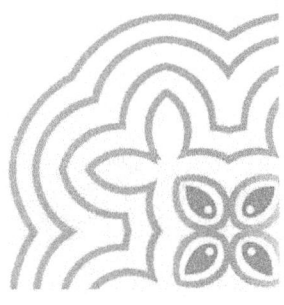

Class Sequence Worksheet

Theme: _____

Quote/Inspiration: _____

Centering/Breathing: _____ **min:** Typically, a pose such as Mountain to get the class started. Other suggestions include Child's Pose or Easy Seated. Commonly, the breathing at this point in class is just having students bring awareness to their breathing/deeper breathing.

Pose(s)	Verbiage/Notes

Active Practicing: _____ **min:** This section would include Sun Salutations, Standing poses and any variations you create.

Pose(s)	Verbiage/Notes

Focusing: _____ **min:** This includes balancing postures, standing and arm balances.

Pose(s)	Verbiage/Notes

Deeper Stretching: _____ min: Floor work, from backbends to stretching forward folds.

Pose(s)	Verbiage/Notes

Relaxing/Meditating: _____ min: Any posture/activity after Savasana such as Easy Seated – and may include visualization or Pranayama.

Pose(s)	Verbiage/Notes

Teacher Notes: How did this sequence work in class?

Class Sequence Worksheet

Theme: _____

Quote/Inspiration: _____

Centering/Breathing: _____ min: Typically, a pose such as Mountain to get the class started. Other suggestions include Child's Pose or Easy Seated. Commonly, the breathing at this point in class is just having students bring awareness to their breathing/deeper breathing.

Pose(s)	Verbiage/Notes

Active Practicing: _____ min: This section would include Sun Salutations, Standing poses and any variations you create.

Pose(s)	Verbiage/Notes

Focusing: _____ min: This includes balancing postures, standing and arm balances.

Pose(s)	Verbiage/Notes

Deeper Stretching: _____ min: Floor work, from backbends to stretching forward folds.

Pose(s)	Verbiage/Notes

Relaxing/Meditating: _____ min: Any posture/activity after Savasana such as Easy Seated – and may include visualization or Pranayama.

Pose(s)	Verbiage/Notes

Teacher Notes: How did this sequence work in class?

Class Sequence Worksheet

Theme: _____

Quote/Inspiration: _____

Centering/Breathing: _____ **min:** Typically, a pose such as Mountain to get the class started. Other suggestions include Child's Pose or Easy Seated. Commonly, the breathing at this point in class is just having students bring awareness to their breathing/deeper breathing.

Pose(s)	Verbiage/Notes

Active Practicing: _____ **min:** This section would include Sun Salutations, Standing poses and any variations you create.

Pose(s)	Verbiage/Notes

Focusing: _____ **min:** This includes balancing postures, standing and arm balances.

Pose(s)	Verbiage/Notes

Deeper Stretching: _____ **min:** Floor work, from backbends to stretching forward folds.

Pose(s)	Verbiage/Notes

Relaxing/Meditating: _____ **min:** Any posture/activity after Savasana such as Easy Seated – and may include visualization or Pranayama.

Pose(s)	Verbiage/Notes

Teacher Notes: How did this sequence work in class?

Class Sequence Worksheet

Theme: _____

Quote/Inspiration: _____

Centering/Breathing: _____ min: Typically, a pose such as Mountain to get the class started. Other suggestions include Child's Pose or Easy Seated. Commonly, the breathing at this point in class is just having students bring awareness to their breathing/deeper breathing.

Pose(s)	Verbiage/Notes

Active Practicing: _____ min: This section would include Sun Salutations, Standing poses and any variations you create.

Pose(s)	Verbiage/Notes

Focusing: _____ min: This includes balancing postures, standing and arm balances.

Pose(s)	Verbiage/Notes

Deeper Stretching: _____ min: Floor work, from backbends to stretching forward folds.

Pose(s)	Verbiage/Notes

Relaxing/Meditating: _____ min: Any posture/activity after Savasana such as Easy Seated – and may include visualization or Pranayama.

Pose(s)	Verbiage/Notes

Teacher Notes: How did this sequence work in class?

Class Sequence Worksheet

Theme: _____

Quote/Inspiration: _____

Centering/Breathing: _____min: Typically, a pose such as Mountain to get the class started. Other suggestions include Child's Pose or Easy Seated. Commonly, the breathing at this point in class is just having students bring awareness to their breathing/deeper breathing.

Pose(s)	Verbiage/Notes

Active Practicing: _____min: This section would include Sun Salutations, Standing poses and any variations you create.

Pose(s)	Verbiage/Notes

Focusing: _____min: This includes balancing postures, standing and arm balances.

Pose(s)	Verbiage/Notes

Deeper Stretching: _____min: Floor work, from backbends to stretching forward folds.

Pose(s)	Verbiage/Notes

Relaxing/Meditating: _____min: Any posture/activity after Savasana such as Easy Seated – and may include visualization or Pranayama.

Pose(s)	Verbiage/Notes

Teacher Notes: How did this sequence work in class?

Class Sequence Worksheet

Theme: _____

Quote/Inspiration: _____

Centering/Breathing: _____ **min:** Typically, a pose such as Mountain to get the class started. Other suggestions include Child's Pose or Easy Seated. Commonly, the breathing at this point in class is just having students bring awareness to their breathing/deeper breathing.

Pose(s)	Verbiage/Notes

Active Practicing: _____ **min:** This section would include Sun Salutations, Standing poses and any variations you create.

Pose(s)	Verbiage/Notes

Focusing: _____ **min:** This includes balancing postures, standing and arm balances.

Pose(s)	Verbiage/Notes

Deeper Stretching: _____ min: Floor work, from backbends to stretching forward folds.

Pose(s)	Verbiage/Notes

Relaxing/Meditating: _____ min: Any posture/activity after Savasana such as Easy Seated – and may include visualization or Pranayama.

Pose(s)	Verbiage/Notes

Teacher Notes: How did this sequence work in class?

Class Sequence Worksheet

Theme: _____

Quote/Inspiration: _____

Centering/Breathing: _____ **min:** Typically, a pose such as Mountain to get the class started. Other suggestions include Child's Pose or Easy Seated. Commonly, the breathing at this point in class is just having students bring awareness to their breathing/deeper breathing.

Pose(s)	Verbiage/Notes

Active Practicing: _____ **min:** This section would include Sun Salutations, Standing poses and any variations you create.

Pose(s)	Verbiage/Notes

Focusing: _____ **min:** This includes balancing postures, standing and arm balances.

Pose(s)	Verbiage/Notes

Deeper Stretching: _____ **min:** Floor work, from backbends to stretching forward folds.

Pose(s)	Verbiage/Notes

Relaxing/Meditating: _____ **min:** Any posture/activity after Savasana such as Easy Seated – and may include visualization or Pranayama.

Pose(s)	Verbiage/Notes

Teacher Notes: How did this sequence work in class?

Class Sequence Worksheet

Theme: _____

Quote/Inspiration: _____

Centering/Breathing: _____ **min:** Typically, a pose such as Mountain to get the class started. Other suggestions include Child's Pose or Easy Seated. Commonly, the breathing at this point in class is just having students bring awareness to their breathing/deeper breathing.

Pose(s)	Verbiage/Notes

Active Practicing: _____ **min:** This section would include Sun Salutations, Standing poses and any variations you create.

Pose(s)	Verbiage/Notes

Focusing: _____ **min:** This includes balancing postures, standing and arm balances.

Pose(s)	Verbiage/Notes

Deeper Stretching: _____**min:** Floor work, from backbends to stretching forward folds.

Pose(s)	Verbiage/Notes

Relaxing/Meditating: _____**min:** Any posture/activity after Savasana such as Easy Seated – and may include visualization or Pranayama.

Pose(s)	Verbiage/Notes

Teacher Notes: How did this sequence work in class?

Class Sequence Worksheet

Theme: _____

Quote/Inspiration: _____

Centering/Breathing: _____ **min:** Typically, a pose such as Mountain to get the class started. Other suggestions include Child's Pose or Easy Seated. Commonly, the breathing at this point in class is just having students bring awareness to their breathing/deeper breathing.

Pose(s)	Verbiage/Notes

Active Practicing: _____ **min:** This section would include Sun Salutations, Standing poses and any variations you create.

Pose(s)	Verbiage/Notes

Focusing: _____ **min:** This includes balancing postures, standing and arm balances.

Pose(s)	Verbiage/Notes

Deeper Stretching: _____ min: Floor work, from backbends to stretching forward folds.

Pose(s)	Verbiage/Notes

Relaxing/Meditating: _____ min: Any posture/activity after Savasana such as Easy Seated – and may include visualization or Pranayama.

Pose(s)	Verbiage/Notes

Teacher Notes: How did this sequence work in class?

Class Sequence Worksheet

Theme: _____

Quote/Inspiration: _____

Centering/Breathing: _____ **min:** Typically, a pose such as Mountain to get the class started. Other suggestions include Child's Pose or Easy Seated. Commonly, the breathing at this point in class is just having students bring awareness to their breathing/deeper breathing.

Pose(s)	Verbiage/Notes

Active Practicing: _____ **min:** This section would include Sun Salutations, Standing poses and any variations you create.

Pose(s)	Verbiage/Notes

Focusing: _____ **min:** This includes balancing postures, standing and arm balances.

Pose(s)	Verbiage/Notes

Deeper Stretching: _____ **min:** Floor work, from backbends to stretching forward folds.

Pose(s)	Verbiage/Notes

Relaxing/Meditating: _____ **min:** Any posture/activity after Savasana such as Easy Seated – and may include visualization or Pranayama.

Pose(s)	Verbiage/Notes

Teacher Notes: How did this sequence work in class?

Class Sequence Worksheet

Theme: _____

Quote/Inspiration: _____

Centering/Breathing: _____ min: Typically, a pose such as Mountain to get the class started. Other suggestions include Child's Pose or Easy Seated. Commonly, the breathing at this point in class is just having students bring awareness to their breathing/deeper breathing.

Pose(s)	Verbiage/Notes

Active Practicing: _____ min: This section would include Sun Salutations, Standing poses and any variations you create.

Pose(s)	Verbiage/Notes

Focusing: _____ min: This includes balancing postures, standing and arm balances.

Pose(s)	Verbiage/Notes

Deeper Stretching: _____ min: Floor work, from backbends to stretching forward folds.

Pose(s)	Verbiage/Notes

Relaxing/Meditating: _____ min: Any posture/activity after Savasana such as Easy Seated – and may include visualization or Pranayama.

Pose(s)	Verbiage/Notes

Teacher Notes: How did this sequence work in class?

Class Sequence Worksheet

Theme: _____

Quote/Inspiration: _____

Centering/Breathing: _____ **min:** Typically, a pose such as Mountain to get the class started. Other suggestions include Child's Pose or Easy Seated. Commonly, the breathing at this point in class is just having students bring awareness to their breathing/deeper breathing.

Pose(s)	Verbiage/Notes

Active Practicing: _____ **min:** This section would include Sun Salutations, Standing poses and any variations you create.

Pose(s)	Verbiage/Notes

Focusing: _____ **min:** This includes balancing postures, standing and arm balances.

Pose(s)	Verbiage/Notes

Deeper Stretching: _____ **min:** Floor work, from backbends to stretching forward folds.

Pose(s)	Verbiage/Notes

Relaxing/Meditating: _____ **min:** Any posture/activity after Savasana such as Easy Seated – and may include visualization or Pranayama.

Pose(s)	Verbiage/Notes

Teacher Notes: How did this sequence work in class?

Class Sequence Worksheet

Theme: _____

Quote/Inspiration: _____

Centering/Breathing: _____ **min:** Typically, a pose such as Mountain to get the class started. Other suggestions include Child's Pose or Easy Seated. Commonly, the breathing at this point in class is just having students bring awareness to their breathing/deeper breathing.

Pose(s)	Verbiage/Notes

Active Practicing: _____ **min:** This section would include Sun Salutations, Standing poses and any variations you create.

Pose(s)	Verbiage/Notes

Focusing: _____ **min:** This includes balancing postures, standing and arm balances.

Pose(s)	Verbiage/Notes

Deeper Stretching: _____**min:** Floor work, from backbends to stretching forward folds.

Pose(s)	Verbiage/Notes

Relaxing/Meditating: _____**min:** Any posture/activity after Savasana such as Easy Seated – and may include visualization or Pranayama.

Pose(s)	Verbiage/Notes

Teacher Notes: How did this sequence work in class?

Class Sequence Worksheet

Theme: _____

Quote/Inspiration: _____

Centering/Breathing: _____ min: Typically, a pose such as Mountain to get the class started. Other suggestions include Child's Pose or Easy Seated. Commonly, the breathing at this point in class is just having students bring awareness to their breathing/deeper breathing.

Pose(s)	Verbiage/Notes

Active Practicing: _____ min: This section would include Sun Salutations, Standing poses and any variations you create.

Pose(s)	Verbiage/Notes

Focusing: _____ min: This includes balancing postures, standing and arm balances.

Pose(s)	Verbiage/Notes

Deeper Stretching: _____ **min:** Floor work, from backbends to stretching forward folds.

Pose(s)	Verbiage/Notes

Relaxing/Meditating: _____ **min:** Any posture/activity after Savasana such as Easy Seated – and may include visualization or Pranayama.

Pose(s)	Verbiage/Notes

Teacher Notes: How did this sequence work in class?

Class Sequence Worksheet

Theme: _____

Quote/Inspiration: _____

Centering/Breathing: _____ **min:** Typically, a pose such as Mountain to get the class started. Other suggestions include Child's Pose or Easy Seated. Commonly, the breathing at this point in class is just having students bring awareness to their breathing/deeper breathing.

Pose(s)	Verbiage/Notes

Active Practicing: _____ **min:** This section would include Sun Salutations, Standing poses and any variations you create.

Pose(s)	Verbiage/Notes

Focusing: _____ **min:** This includes balancing postures, standing and arm balances.

Pose(s)	Verbiage/Notes

Deeper Stretching: _____ **min:** Floor work, from backbends to stretching forward folds.

Pose(s)	Verbiage/Notes

Relaxing/Meditating: _____ **min:** Any posture/activity after Savasana such as Easy Seated – and may include visualization or Pranayama.

Pose(s)	Verbiage/Notes

Teacher Notes: How did this sequence work in class?

Class Sequence Worksheet

Theme: _____

Quote/Inspiration: _____

Centering/Breathing: _____ **min:** Typically, a pose such as Mountain to get the class started. Other suggestions include Child's Pose or Easy Seated. Commonly, the breathing at this point in class is just having students bring awareness to their breathing/deeper breathing.

Pose(s)	Verbiage/Notes

Active Practicing: _____ **min:** This section would include Sun Salutations, Standing poses and any variations you create.

Pose(s)	Verbiage/Notes

Focusing: _____ **min:** This includes balancing postures, standing and arm balances.

Pose(s)	Verbiage/Notes

Deeper Stretching: _____**min:** Floor work, from backbends to stretching forward folds.

Pose(s)	Verbiage/Notes

Relaxing/Meditating: _____**min:** Any posture/activity after Savasana such as Easy Seated – and may include visualization or Pranayama.

Pose(s)	Verbiage/Notes

Teacher Notes: How did this sequence work in class?

Class Sequence Worksheet

Theme: _____

Quote/Inspiration: _____

Centering/Breathing: _____ **min:** Typically, a pose such as Mountain to get the class started. Other suggestions include Child's Pose or Easy Seated. Commonly, the breathing at this point in class is just having students bring awareness to their breathing/deeper breathing.

Pose(s)	Verbiage/Notes

Active Practicing: _____ **min:** This section would include Sun Salutations, Standing poses and any variations you create.

Pose(s)	Verbiage/Notes

Focusing: _____ **min:** This includes balancing postures, standing and arm balances.

Pose(s)	Verbiage/Notes

Deeper Stretching: _____**min:** Floor work, from backbends to stretching forward folds.

Pose(s)	Verbiage/Notes

Relaxing/Meditating: _____**min:** Any posture/activity after Savasana such as Easy Seated – and may include visualization or Pranayama.

Pose(s)	Verbiage/Notes

Teacher Notes: How did this sequence work in class?

Class Sequence Worksheet

Theme: _____

Quote/Inspiration: _____

Centering/Breathing: _____ **min:** Typically, a pose such as Mountain to get the class started. Other suggestions include Child's Pose or Easy Seated. Commonly, the breathing at this point in class is just having students bring awareness to their breathing/deeper breathing.

Pose(s)	Verbiage/Notes

Active Practicing: _____ **min:** This section would include Sun Salutations, Standing poses and any variations you create.

Pose(s)	Verbiage/Notes

Focusing: _____ **min:** This includes balancing postures, standing and arm balances.

Pose(s)	Verbiage/Notes

Deeper Stretching: _____ min: Floor work, from backbends to stretching forward folds.

Pose(s)	Verbiage/Notes

Relaxing/Meditating: _____ min: Any posture/activity after Savasana such as Easy Seated – and may include visualization or Pranayama.

Pose(s)	Verbiage/Notes

Teacher Notes: How did this sequence work in class?

Class Sequence Worksheet

Theme: _____

Quote/Inspiration: _____

Centering/Breathing: _____ **min:** Typically, a pose such as Mountain to get the class started. Other suggestions include Child's Pose or Easy Seated. Commonly, the breathing at this point in class is just having students bring awareness to their breathing/deeper breathing.

Pose(s)	Verbiage/Notes

Active Practicing: _____ **min:** This section would include Sun Salutations, Standing poses and any variations you create.

Pose(s)	Verbiage/Notes

Focusing: _____ **min:** This includes balancing postures, standing and arm balances.

Pose(s)	Verbiage/Notes

Deeper Stretching: _____ min: Floor work, from backbends to stretching forward folds.

Pose(s)	Verbiage/Notes

Relaxing/Meditating: _____ min: Any posture/activity after Savasana such as Easy Seated – and may include visualization or Pranayama.

Pose(s)	Verbiage/Notes

Teacher Notes: How did this sequence work in class?

Class Sequence Worksheet

Theme: _____

Quote/Inspiration: _____

Centering/Breathing: _____min: Typically, a pose such as Mountain to get the class started. Other suggestions include Child's Pose or Easy Seated. Commonly, the breathing at this point in class is just having students bring awareness to their breathing/deeper breathing.

Pose(s)	Verbiage/Notes

Active Practicing: _____min: This section would include Sun Salutations, Standing poses and any variations you create.

Pose(s)	Verbiage/Notes

Focusing: _____min: This includes balancing postures, standing and arm balances.

Pose(s)	Verbiage/Notes

Deeper Stretching: _____ min: Floor work, from backbends to stretching forward folds.

Pose(s)	Verbiage/Notes

Relaxing/Meditating: _____ min: Any posture/activity after Savasana such as Easy Seated – and may include visualization or Pranayama.

Pose(s)	Verbiage/Notes

Teacher Notes: How did this sequence work in class?

Works Cited in this Guide

Baptiste, B. (2002). *Journey Into Power.* New York: Fireside.

Desikachar, T. (1995, 1999). *The Heart of Yoga, Developing a Personal Practice.* Rochester: Innter Traditions International.

Stephens, M. (2010). *Teaching Yoga, Essential Foundations and Techniques.* Berkeley: North Atlantic Books.

Stephens, M. (2012). *Yoga Sequencing, Designing Transformative Yoga Classes.* Berkeley: North Atlantic Books.

And years of teaching yoga! 😊